Chapter 1: Understanding Chickenpox

What is Chickenpox?

Chickenpox, medically known as varicella, is a highly contagious viral infection caused by the varicella-zoster virus. It primarily affects children but can also occur in adults who have not previously contracted the disease or been vaccinated. Characterized by an itchy rash that develops into fluid-filled blisters, chickenpox is often accompanied by fever, fatigue, and loss of appetite. The rash typically appears in waves, beginning on the face, chest, and back before spreading to the rest of the body. Understanding the signs and symptoms of chickenpox is essential for parents to recognize the condition early and manage their child's health effectively.

The transmission of chickenpox occurs through respiratory droplets when an infected person coughs or sneezes, as well as through direct contact with the blisters. The virus is particularly contagious, and individuals are considered infectious from about two days before the rash appears until all blisters have crusted over. Vaccination is the most effective way to prevent chickenpox. The varicella vaccine, which is typically administered to children at 12-15 months of age, significantly reduces the chances of contracting the virus. For those who do develop chickenpox despite vaccination, the symptoms are usually milder and the duration shorter.

Parents should also be aware of the differences in chickenpox presentation between children and adults. While children often experience a mild illness with fewer complications, adults are at a higher risk for severe symptoms and complications, such as pneumonia or encephalitis. Therefore, it is crucial for parents to ensure that their children are vaccinated, not only for their protection but also to prevent the spread of the virus to others, particularly vulnerable populations such as newborns or immunocompromised individuals.

In addition to vaccination, various home remedies can help alleviate the discomfort caused by chickenpox symptoms. Oatmeal baths, calamine lotion, and antihistamines may provide relief from itching and irritation. It is essential to keep the child's nails trimmed to prevent scratching, which can lead to secondary infections. Monitoring for any complications, such as bacterial infections of the skin or respiratory issues, is also vital during the recovery phase. Parents should maintain communication with their healthcare provider to ensure that any concerning symptoms are addressed promptly.

Myths and misconceptions surrounding chickenpox can lead to confusion and misinformation among parents. For example, some believe that chickenpox is a benign childhood illness that poses no significant threat, while others may fear the vaccine's safety. Understanding the history and evolution of the chickenpox vaccine can help dispel these myths and reassure parents about vaccination's importance. Additionally, recognizing the relationship between chickenpox and shingles, which can occur later in life after a chickenpox infection, highlights the long-term implications of the virus. Comprehensive knowledge about chickenpox empowers parents to make informed decisions regarding prevention, care, and overall health for their children.

Symptoms and Diagnosis

Chickenpox, caused by the varicella-zoster virus, is characterized by a distinct set of symptoms that typically begin with mild flu-like signs before the characteristic rash appears. Initially, children may experience a low-grade fever, fatigue, loss of appetite, and headache. These early symptoms can often be mistaken for other viral infections, making it crucial for parents to stay vigilant. Within 1 to 2 days of the onset of these symptoms, the signature itchy rash emerges, starting as small red spots that quickly develop into fluid-filled blisters. This progression is a key indicator of chickenpox, and understanding these symptoms can help parents identify the illness early.

Diagnosing chickenpox is largely based on the clinical presentation of the rash and accompanying symptoms. Healthcare providers typically confirm the diagnosis through visual examination, taking into account the pattern and progression of the rash. In some cases, especially when the symptoms are atypical or in adults, laboratory tests may be employed to detect the varicella-zoster virus. It's essential for parents to consult a healthcare professional if they suspect their child has chickenpox, particularly if the child is immunocompromised, as the disease can lead to more severe complications in these cases.

For parents seeking to manage the symptoms of chickenpox at home, several remedies can help alleviate discomfort. Calamine lotion and oatmeal baths are popular options for soothing itching and skin irritation. Over-the-counter antihistamines may also provide relief from itching, while acetaminophen can help reduce fever. It is important to avoid giving aspirin to children with chickenpox, as it has been linked to Reye's syndrome, a rare but serious condition. Parents should also encourage their child to avoid scratching the blisters to reduce the risk of secondary infections.

The impact of chickenpox can vary significantly between children and adults. While chickenpox is generally mild in children, adults are at a higher risk for severe complications, including pneumonia and encephalitis. Pregnant women who contract chickenpox, particularly in the first or second trimester, face additional risks, including potential birth defects and complications for the newborn. Therefore, it is vital for parents to understand these differences and to seek medical advice promptly if they suspect exposure to the virus, especially in vulnerable populations.

In the realm of prevention, the varicella vaccine has played a crucial role in mitigating the incidence of chickenpox. The vaccine is recommended for children, with the first dose typically administered between 12 and 15 months of age and a second dose between 4 and 6 years. Understanding the history and evolution of the chickenpox vaccine can empower parents to make informed choices about vaccination for their children. Moreover, recognizing that chickenpox can later manifest as shingles in adults reinforces the importance of preventative measures, not only for individual health but also for public health as a whole.

Chapter 2: Chickenpox Prevention and Vaccination

The Importance of Vaccination

Vaccination plays a crucial role in preventing chickenpox, a highly contagious viral infection that can have serious implications for children and adults alike. The chickenpox vaccine, introduced in the mid-1990s, has significantly reduced the incidence of this disease. By immunizing children, families not only protect their own loved ones but also contribute to community immunity, reducing the chances of outbreaks and protecting those who are unable to be vaccinated due to medical reasons. Understanding the importance of vaccination is essential for parents seeking to safeguard their children's health and well-being.

One of the most compelling reasons for vaccinating against chickenpox is the prevention of severe illness and complications. While chickenpox is often viewed as a mild childhood disease, it can lead to serious complications such as pneumonia, encephalitis, and secondary bacterial infections. Adults are particularly at risk for more severe manifestations of the disease, which can lead to hospitalization. By ensuring that children receive the vaccine, parents can significantly decrease the likelihood of these serious health outcomes, allowing their children to grow up healthier and more resilient.

In addition to protecting individual health, vaccination against chickenpox is vital for those who are immunocompromised or pregnant. For individuals with weakened immune systems, chickenpox can be life-threatening. The vaccine helps prevent the spread of the virus, thereby protecting vulnerable populations who may not have the same immunity as healthy individuals. Furthermore, pregnant women who contract chickenpox are at risk for serious complications that can affect both the mother and the developing fetus. Vaccination prior to pregnancy can help mitigate these risks, fostering a safer environment for both mother and child.

Moreover, the history and evolution of the chickenpox vaccine highlight its effectiveness and the significant strides made in public health. Initially introduced as a single-dose vaccine, the recommendations have evolved to encourage a two-dose schedule, which provides even stronger immunity. This evolution reflects ongoing research and the commitment of health organizations to enhance protection against chickenpox. By understanding how the vaccine has developed over time, parents can appreciate the advances in medical science that have led to safer and more effective preventive measures.

Finally, it is essential to address common myths and misconceptions surrounding the chickenpox vaccine. Some parents may fear that vaccination could lead to the disease itself or cause adverse effects. However, the reality is that the vaccine contains a weakened form of the virus, which stimulates the immune system without causing the full-blown disease. Education about the benefits and safety of vaccination is vital for dispelling these myths and ensuring that parents feel confident in their choices. By prioritizing vaccination, parents not only protect their children but also contribute to the health and safety of their communities.

Vaccination Schedule for Children

Vaccination is a crucial aspect of protecting children from chickenpox, a highly contagious viral infection that can lead to serious complications. The chickenpox vaccine, known as varicella vaccine, is typically administered in two doses. The first dose is given to children between 12 to 15 months of age, while the second dose is recommended between 4 to 6 years of age. This schedule ensures that children develop adequate immunity to the varicella-zoster virus, reducing the risk of contracting chickenpox and its potential complications later in life.

Parents should be aware of the importance of adhering to the vaccination schedule to maximize protection. The varicella vaccine is highly effective, with studies showing that it reduces the incidence of chickenpox by about 90% among vaccinated individuals. Additionally, for those who may still contract the virus post-vaccination, the symptoms are typically milder, with fewer lesions and a shorter duration of illness. This highlights the vaccine's role not only in prevention but also in mitigating the severity of the disease.

It is essential for parents to keep track of their child's vaccination records and consult with their pediatricians regarding any missed doses. If a child has not received the vaccine within the recommended age range, it is advisable to catch up as soon as possible. The vaccine can be administered at any age, and it is never too late to protect a child from chickenpox. Furthermore, health care providers may recommend the vaccine for older children and adults who have not previously been vaccinated or have not had chickenpox.

In addition to the routine vaccination schedule, parents should also be aware of the specific considerations for immunocompromised children. For these children, live vaccines like the varicella vaccine may not be appropriate due to their weakened immune systems. Therefore, families should discuss alternative preventive measures with their healthcare provider, including passive immunization methods, to ensure that these vulnerable children receive adequate protection against chickenpox.

Understanding the vaccination schedule and its importance is vital for all parents. Keeping informed about the chickenpox vaccine, its efficacy, and the potential risks associated with the disease can empower parents to make educated decisions regarding their child's health. As the varicella vaccine continues to play a significant role in public health, timely vaccinations contribute to community immunity, protecting not only individual children but also those who are unable to be vaccinated due to medical reasons.

Chickenpox Vaccine Effectiveness

The effectiveness of the chickenpox vaccine has been a significant advancement in public health, greatly reducing the incidence and severity of chickenpox infections. The varicella vaccine, introduced in the mid-1990s, is approximately 90% effective at preventing chickenpox after two doses. For parents, this means that by vaccinating their children, they are not only protecting them from the itchy rash and discomfort associated with the illness but also from potential complications such as pneumonia or bacterial infections that can arise from chickenpox.

Vaccination has also contributed to herd immunity, which protects those who cannot be vaccinated due to medical reasons, such as immunocompromised individuals. When a large portion of the population is vaccinated, the spread of the virus is significantly limited, reducing the chances of outbreaks. This is particularly important for communities with vulnerable individuals, including infants, pregnant women, and those undergoing treatments that weaken the immune system. Parents can feel reassured that by vaccinating their children, they are playing an essential role in safeguarding their entire community.

Despite the vaccine's high effectiveness, breakthrough infections can occur, though they tend to be less severe than cases in unvaccinated individuals. These milder cases often present with fewer lesions and a shorter duration of symptoms. Parents should understand that while the vaccine greatly reduces the risk of severe illness, it does not confer absolute immunity. Therefore, continued awareness of chickenpox symptoms and appropriate care is necessary, even for vaccinated children.

Research has shown that the long-term effectiveness of the chickenpox vaccine remains robust, with studies indicating that immunity persists for many years after vaccination. However, it is still essential for parents to ensure their children receive the recommended two doses, which are typically administered at ages 12-15 months and 4-6 years. This two-dose schedule maximizes protection and contributes to the overall decline in chickenpox cases and related complications.

It is also crucial for parents to be aware of the relationship between chickenpox and shingles, especially in vaccinated individuals. The varicella vaccine not only protects against chickenpox but also reduces the risk of developing shingles later in life. Understanding this connection can help parents make informed decisions regarding vaccinations and the long-term health of their children. Overall, the chickenpox vaccine represents a vital tool in preventing illness and protecting both individual and public health.

Chapter 3: Home Remedies for Chickenpox Symptoms

Soothing Itchy Skin

Soothing itchy skin during a chickenpox infection is essential for ensuring comfort and preventing further complications. The intense itching associated with chickenpox can be distressing for both children and parents. To help alleviate this discomfort, various methods are available that cater to different age groups and sensitivities. Parents should prioritize gentle approaches and be cautious about using harsh chemicals or treatments that could exacerbate the skin irritation.

One of the simplest and most effective remedies involves maintaining cool skin. Keeping the environment cool can help minimize itching. Parents can dress their children in loose, breathable clothing and use lightweight bedding. Frequent cool baths can also provide temporary relief. Adding colloidal oatmeal or baking soda to the bath water can enhance the soothing effect, allowing the child to soak for a while to relieve the itchy sensation. After bathing, it is essential to pat the skin dry gently rather than rubbing it, as this can further irritate the blisters.

Over-the-counter antihistamines can be beneficial in managing itching, especially for older children and adults. These medications can help reduce the body's allergic response and provide a calming effect on the skin. However, it is crucial to consult with a healthcare provider before administering any medication, particularly to young children. In some cases, topical treatments like calamine lotion can also offer relief by providing a cooling sensation and drying out blisters, but they should be applied with care to avoid further irritation.

Natural remedies can also be effective for soothing itchy skin. Aloe vera gel is renowned for its skin-healing properties and can be applied directly to the affected areas. Chamomile and lavender essential oils, when diluted with a carrier oil, can provide a calming effect and might help to relieve itching. Parents should ensure that no allergies to these natural remedies exist before application. It is essential to monitor the child's reaction to any new treatment, as individual sensitivities can vary significantly.

Lastly, maintaining proper skin hygiene is crucial during a chickenpox infection. Keeping the blisters clean and preventing them from becoming infected is vital for recovery. Parents should gently wash the affected areas with mild soap and water, ensuring that any crusts are not picked, which can lead to scarring or secondary infections. By combining these strategies, parents can significantly improve their child's comfort level and support a smoother recovery process from chickenpox.

Managing Fever and Discomfort

Managing fever and discomfort during a chickenpox infection is crucial for ensuring a smoother recovery for your child. Fever is a common symptom associated with chickenpox, often appearing as the body fights off the varicella virus. In most cases, this fever is mild to moderate, but it can cause significant discomfort. Parents should monitor their child's temperature regularly and be prepared to take appropriate steps to alleviate discomfort. Over-the-counter medications, such as acetaminophen, can help reduce fever and relieve discomfort, but it's essential to avoid aspirin due to the risk of Reye's syndrome, especially in children.

In addition to fever management, addressing skin discomfort caused by chickenpox lesions is vital. The itchy, blister-like rashes can lead to excessive scratching, which may result in secondary infections. To manage this discomfort, parents can apply calamine lotion or anti-itch creams containing ingredients like hydrocortisone to soothe the skin. Keeping your child's nails short and clean can help minimize the risk of scratching. Additionally, using cool compresses can provide temporary relief from itching and promote comfort.

Hydration plays a significant role in managing fever and overall discomfort during a chickenpox infection. Children may be reluctant to drink fluids due to fever or mouth sores caused by the virus. Offering frequent sips of water, clear broths, or electrolyte solutions can help keep your child hydrated. Ice chips or popsicles may also be appealing and provide both hydration and relief from fever. Keeping your child well-hydrated is essential not only for comfort but also for supporting their immune system as it fights off the infection.

Creating a comfortable environment is another important aspect of managing discomfort during chickenpox. Ensure that your child is dressed in loose, breathable clothing to prevent irritation of the skin. Keeping the room cool and well-ventilated can help reduce fever and promote comfort. Encourage your child to rest and engage in calming activities, such as reading or watching movies, to distract them from discomfort. A peaceful environment can significantly aid in their emotional well-being during this time.

Finally, while managing fever and discomfort at home is often effective, it's crucial to recognize when to seek medical attention. If your child's fever persists for more than a few days, becomes exceptionally high, or is accompanied by other concerning symptoms such as difficulty breathing or severe headache, consult your healthcare provider. Being proactive about your child's health during a chickenpox infection can help prevent complications and ensure a smoother recovery. With appropriate care and attention, managing fever and discomfort can lead to a more positive experience for both parents and children alike.

Hydration and Nutrition

Hydration and nutrition play crucial roles in managing chickenpox, not only in alleviating symptoms but also in aiding recovery. When a child contracts chickenpox, the body expends energy fighting off the virus, leading to an increased need for fluids and essential nutrients. Parents should ensure that their child stays well-hydrated, as fever and skin lesions can lead to dehydration. Water, clear broths, and electrolyte solutions can help maintain hydration levels. Additionally, offering soft foods that are easy to swallow can be beneficial, especially if the child has mouth sores due to the infection.

In terms of nutrition, a well-balanced diet rich in vitamins and minerals can support the immune system during the recovery process. Foods high in vitamin C, such as fruits and vegetables, can help boost immunity and promote healing. Protein is also essential, as it aids in tissue repair and recovery. Incorporating lean meats, dairy, and legumes into meals can provide the necessary building blocks for the body to recover effectively. Parents should be mindful to avoid overly spicy or acidic foods that might irritate mouth sores.

For children experiencing severe itching due to chickenpox, certain home remedies can complement hydration and nutrition. Oatmeal baths and topical applications of calamine lotion can soothe the skin and reduce discomfort. These remedies, along with adequate fluid intake and nutritious meals, can help create a comfortable environment for healing. Ensuring that the child is relaxed and not overly stressed will also contribute to their overall well-being during the infection.

It is particularly important for parents to monitor the nutritional needs of children with chickenpox, especially those who may have additional health concerns. Immunocompromised individuals may face more significant challenges in both hydration and nutrition due to the heightened risk of complications. These children may require specialized dietary interventions to ensure they are receiving adequate nutrients while managing their symptoms. Consulting with a healthcare professional can provide tailored advice for these situations.

In summary, hydration and nutrition are foundational elements in the management of chickenpox. By keeping children well-hydrated and providing a balanced diet rich in essential nutrients, parents can support their recovery and minimize discomfort. Addressing these needs not only helps in managing the immediate symptoms of chickenpox but also fosters a stronger immune response, paving the way for a smoother recovery process.

Chapter 4: Chickenpox in Adults vs. Children

Symptoms in Adults

Symptoms of chickenpox in adults can be more severe than in children, making it crucial for parents to be informed about what to look for if their child shows signs of infection. The initial symptoms typically appear between 10 to 21 days after exposure to the virus. Adults may experience a range of symptoms that include fever, fatigue, headache, and loss of appetite. These pre-rash symptoms can last for one to two days and serve as an early indicator that the body is fighting off the varicella-zoster virus.

The hallmark of chickenpox is the characteristic rash, which usually begins as small red spots that rapidly develop into itchy blisters filled with fluid. In adults, this rash can cover a larger area of the body and may appear in clusters or patches. The blisters eventually crust over, forming scabs, which can take a week or more to heal. Parents should monitor their children closely during this phase, as the intense itching can lead to scratching and potential secondary infections.

In addition to the common symptoms, adults may experience more severe complications from chickenpox, such as pneumonia or encephalitis. These complications are relatively rare but can be serious, especially in adults who are pregnant, have weakened immune systems, or have pre-existing health conditions. Parents must be vigilant and seek medical attention if their child exhibits difficulty breathing, confusion, or persistent high fever, as these may be signs of complications requiring immediate care.

It is also important to note that symptoms can vary significantly between children and adults. While children often recover without serious issues, adults may experience a more prolonged illness and a higher risk of complications. Parents should educate themselves about the differences in symptom severity and be prepared to adjust their care approach accordingly. This knowledge can help in identifying when home remedies might be sufficient and when medical intervention is necessary.

Lastly, understanding common myths surrounding chickenpox can empower parents to respond effectively to symptoms. Many believe that chickenpox is a mild childhood illness, but the reality is that it can pose serious risks for adults and certain vulnerable populations. By recognizing the symptoms and being informed about the potential complications, parents can play a pivotal role in the effective management and recovery of their child's chickenpox infection.

Complications in Adults

Complications from chickenpox in adults can be more severe than in children, and understanding these risks is crucial for parents, especially those with older children or other family members who may be susceptible. While chickenpox is typically a mild illness in children, adults face a higher likelihood of developing complications such as pneumonia, encephalitis, and secondary bacterial infections. These conditions can lead to more serious health issues, requiring medical intervention and sometimes hospitalization. It is essential for parents to recognize the potential for these complications to ensure timely care and support for their loved ones.

Pneumonia is one of the most common complications associated with chickenpox in adults, occurring in approximately 10 to 20 percent of cases. This respiratory condition can develop when the varicella-zoster virus infects the lungs, leading to symptoms such as difficulty breathing, chest pain, and a persistent cough. Parents should be aware of these symptoms and seek immediate medical attention if they occur, as pneumonia can progress rapidly and may require treatment with antiviral medications or hospitalization for severe cases.

Another significant concern is the risk of encephalitis, which is inflammation of the brain. While rare, this serious complication can lead to neurological issues, including seizures, confusion, and in some cases, long-term disabilities. The symptoms of encephalitis may not appear until a few days after the rash develops, making it essential for parents to monitor their loved ones closely during the course of the illness. If any neurological symptoms arise, prompt medical evaluation is crucial to mitigate potential long-term effects.

In addition to these severe complications, adults with chickenpox are also at risk for secondary bacterial infections, particularly when scratching the itchy blisters. These infections can occur in the skin, leading to cellulitis or abscesses, and may require antibiotic treatment. Parents should emphasize the importance of keeping the affected areas clean and avoiding scratching to minimize this risk. Utilizing home remedies such as oatmeal baths and calamine lotion can help soothe itching and reduce the likelihood of secondary infections.

Finally, it is important for parents to be aware of the implications of chickenpox in the context of pregnancy. Pregnant women who contract chickenpox are at risk for serious complications, and the virus can also affect the unborn child, leading to congenital varicella syndrome. Understanding these risks underscores the importance of vaccination and prevention strategies for both children and adults. By staying informed and vigilant, parents can better manage the potential complications of chickenpox and ensure that their families remain healthy and safe.

Recovery Differences

Recovery from chickenpox can vary significantly between children and adults, primarily due to differences in immune response and overall health. In children, chickenpox typically presents as a mild illness characterized by fever and an itchy rash that progresses through various stages. Most children recover within one to two weeks, experiencing only mild discomfort. The immune system of children is generally robust, enabling them to combat the varicella-zoster virus effectively. In contrast, adults tend to experience more severe symptoms and a longer recovery period. Adult cases are frequently accompanied by higher fever, more extensive rash coverage, and a greater likelihood of complications, such as pneumonia or bacterial infections, which can prolong the healing process.

Understanding the nuances of recovery is essential for parents, especially when considering the potential for complications. In children, while the risk of severe complications is low, children with weakened immune systems or underlying health conditions may face a more challenging recovery. For adults, the increased risk of complications means that the recovery process may require more vigilant monitoring and care. Parents should be aware of the symptoms that warrant medical attention, such as difficulty breathing, persistent high fever, or rash that appears infected. This understanding can help parents navigate the recovery phase more effectively and ensure that their child receives appropriate care if complications arise.

Home remedies can play a significant role in alleviating symptoms and promoting comfort during recovery. Parents are encouraged to utilize soothing baths with colloidal oatmeal, apply calamine lotion to itchy spots, and maintain hydration to ease fever and discomfort. These remedies can provide relief and help manage the symptoms associated with chickenpox, making the recovery experience more bearable for both children and adults. It is essential, however, to consult with a healthcare professional before using any home remedies, especially when treating adults or immunocompromised individuals, as their needs may differ significantly.

Post-infection care is another critical aspect of recovery. For children, it is important to monitor for any signs of secondary infections, particularly in areas where scratching may have occurred. Keeping the child's nails trimmed and encouraging them to wear gloves can help minimize skin damage and reduce the risk of infection. Adults, on the other hand, should be attentive to lingering symptoms such as fatigue or respiratory issues, which may require follow-up care. Additionally, parents should be aware of the potential for shingles, a reactivation of the varicella-zoster virus, which can occur later in life after recovering from chickenpox. This knowledge can help in managing long-term health considerations.

Finally, addressing myths and misconceptions surrounding chickenpox recovery can empower parents with accurate information. Common myths, such as the belief that chickenpox guarantees lifelong immunity, can lead to complacency regarding vaccination and prevention. Understanding that the varicella vaccine significantly reduces the severity of chickenpox, even if contracted, is crucial for informed decision-making. Furthermore, recognizing that immunocompromised individuals may experience severe complications from chickenpox underscores the importance of vaccination and preventive measures. By equipping themselves with accurate knowledge, parents can better support their children's recovery and navigate the complexities of chickenpox and its long-term implications.

Chapter 5: Managing Chickenpox Complications

Recognizing Serious Symptoms

Recognizing serious symptoms of chickenpox is crucial for parents to ensure the well-being of their children and to take appropriate action when necessary. While chickenpox is often seen as a mild illness, there are instances where it can lead to serious complications, particularly in certain populations such as infants, adults, and immunocompromised individuals. Parents should be vigilant in monitoring their child's symptoms and understanding when to seek medical attention.

One of the primary symptoms that can indicate a more serious issue is a high fever that persists beyond the usual duration associated with chickenpox. While a mild fever is common, a fever that exceeds 102°F for more than three days may suggest a secondary infection or other complications. Additionally, if a child experiences difficulty breathing, chest pain, or persistent coughing, these could be signs of pneumonia, a rare but serious complication linked to chickenpox.

Another red flag is the development of severe skin infections. The chickenpox rash typically goes through stages, but if the blisters appear swollen, filled with pus, or if a child shows signs of increased pain or tenderness in the affected areas, it may indicate a bacterial infection that requires medical intervention. Parents should also be alert to any signs of spreading rash beyond the typical distribution of chickenpox, as this could signal a more serious condition.

Neurological symptoms should also be taken seriously. If a child exhibits signs of confusion, seizures, or difficulty waking up, these may indicate encephalitis or other neurological complications. Such symptoms require immediate medical evaluation, as they can significantly impact the child's health. Parents should not hesitate to seek emergency care in these situations, as timely intervention can make a critical difference.

Finally, it is essential for parents to be aware of the psychological and emotional toll that chickenpox can take on children, particularly in terms of itching and discomfort. In rare cases, severe itching can lead to excessive scratching, which may cause secondary infections or scarring. Parents should consider using home remedies to alleviate discomfort, but they must also recognize when to consult healthcare professionals if symptoms escalate. Understanding these serious symptoms can empower parents to respond promptly, minimizing risks and ensuring a smoother recovery process for their children.

Treatment Options for Complications

Complications arising from chickenpox can vary in severity and may require specific treatment approaches. One of the most common complications is bacterial superinfection of the skin lesions. Parents should be vigilant for signs of infection, such as increased redness, warmth, swelling, or pus at the site of the chickenpox blisters. If these symptoms occur, a healthcare provider may prescribe antibiotics to address the bacterial infection. It is crucial to follow the prescribed treatment regimen to ensure proper healing and prevent further complications.

Another potential complication of chickenpox is pneumonia, which can be particularly concerning in adults and immunocompromised individuals. Symptoms of pneumonia may include difficulty breathing, persistent cough, chest pain, and high fever. In such cases, immediate medical attention is necessary. Treatment may involve hospitalization, where supportive care such as oxygen therapy and intravenous fluids can be administered. In some instances, antiviral medications may also be prescribed to manage the viral infection more effectively.

Encephalitis, though rare, is a serious complication that can occur after chickenpox. This inflammation of the brain can lead to neurological symptoms such as confusion, seizures, or changes in consciousness. If a child shows any signs of neurological distress following a chickenpox infection, it is essential to seek emergency medical care. Treatment for encephalitis may include hospitalization and supportive therapies, as well as antiviral medications if indicated. Early intervention can significantly improve outcomes.

Parents should also be aware of the risk of dehydration, particularly in younger children who may be reluctant to drink due to mouth sores or fever. Ensuring adequate fluid intake is vital for recovery. In cases of severe dehydration, oral rehydration solutions or intravenous fluids may be necessary. Additionally, fever management is an important aspect of care. Over-the-counter medications such as acetaminophen can help reduce fever and discomfort, but parents should avoid giving aspirin to children due to the risk of Reye's syndrome.

Finally, it is essential for parents to monitor their child's overall recovery process and be aware of any lingering symptoms. Post-infection care may involve ensuring that the child's skin heals properly and addressing any scarring that may occur. Some parents choose to consult dermatologists for advice on minimizing scars. Supportive care, including proper nutrition and rest, can facilitate a smooth recovery. Understanding these treatment options for complications can empower parents to act quickly and effectively, ensuring the best possible outcomes for their children during and after a chickenpox infection.

When to Seek Medical Help

Recognizing when to seek medical help for chickenpox is crucial for ensuring the health and safety of your child. While chickenpox is often considered a mild illness in children, there are certain circumstances where professional medical intervention becomes necessary. Parents should closely monitor the symptoms and understand the warning signs that indicate a potential complication or more serious health issue. If your child experiences difficulty breathing, persistent high fever, or severe itching that does not respond to home remedies, it is essential to contact your healthcare provider promptly.

In addition to the initial symptoms, parents should be vigilant about observing the progression of the rash. If the blisters become infected or show signs of pus, redness, or increased swelling, this could indicate a secondary bacterial infection. In such cases, medical evaluation is important to prevent further complications. Similarly, if your child displays signs of dehydration, such as decreased urination or excessive thirst, this warrants immediate medical attention, as dehydration can exacerbate the condition.

Adults suffering from chickenpox may encounter different challenges than children. While many adults have been vaccinated or previously infected, those who are not immune can face more severe symptoms. If an adult develops chickenpox and experiences severe respiratory symptoms, extreme fatigue, or neurological symptoms like confusion or seizures, they should seek medical help without delay. The risk of complications is higher in adults, and timely intervention can lead to better outcomes.

For pregnant women, chickenpox poses unique risks that require careful monitoring. If a pregnant woman is exposed to the virus or develops chickenpox, it is crucial to consult with a healthcare provider immediately. The virus can affect the developing fetus, leading to potential complications such as congenital varicella syndrome. Early medical evaluation can help manage the risks and provide appropriate care for both mother and baby, including the consideration of antiviral medications if necessary.

Lastly, parents of immunocompromised children should be particularly cautious. Chickenpox can lead to severe complications in children with weakened immune systems, necessitating prompt medical attention at the first sign of infection. Such children may require antiviral treatments and additional supportive care to manage symptoms effectively. By understanding these critical indicators and when to seek help, parents can play a proactive role in managing chickenpox and protecting their family's health.

Chapter 6: Chickenpox and its Impact on Pregnancy

Risks to the Mother

Risks associated with chickenpox during pregnancy can pose significant concerns for expectant mothers. While many parents are aware of the complications that can arise in children, it is essential to understand that pregnant women are at a unique risk when exposed to the varicella-zoster virus. If a mother contracts chickenpox during the first trimester, the potential for congenital varicella syndrome exists, which can lead to severe birth defects, including limb abnormalities, eye issues, and neurological problems. The impact of the virus on fetal development highlights the importance of vaccination and prevention strategies before pregnancy.

Additionally, women who contract chickenpox later in pregnancy, especially in the third trimester, face an increased risk of complications. If a mother develops chickenpox within a week of delivery, her newborn is at risk for neonatal varicella, a severe form of chickenpox that can lead to serious health issues in the infant, including pneumonia and even death. This underscores the importance of ensuring that mothers are immunized against chickenpox prior to conception to minimize risks to both themselves and their unborn children.

Moreover, pregnant women who are immunocompromised or have pre-existing health conditions may be at an even higher risk for severe chickenpox infections. The virus can lead to complications such as pneumonia and hepatitis in these individuals, which can further complicate pregnancy and delivery. It is crucial for these women to consult with healthcare providers to discuss vaccination and preventive measures before becoming pregnant, as their health can significantly influence the course of the pregnancy and the well-being of the baby.

In addition to the physical risks, chickenpox can also have emotional and psychological effects on expectant mothers. The stress and anxiety associated with potential complications can be overwhelming, particularly for first-time parents. Awareness and education about chickenpox and its risks can alleviate some of this stress, empowering mothers to take proactive steps in preventing the virus through vaccination and avoiding exposure during pregnancy.

Ultimately, understanding the risks of chickenpox during pregnancy is vital for both the mother and the child. By emphasizing vaccination and making informed choices about prevention, parents can protect themselves and their future children from the potential dangers associated with this virus. Awareness and education are key to ensuring a healthier future for both mothers and their newborns.

Potential Effects on the Baby

Potential effects of chickenpox on a developing baby can vary significantly depending on the timing of the infection during pregnancy. If a pregnant woman contracts chickenpox, particularly during the first trimester, there is a risk of congenital varicella syndrome. This condition can lead to serious birth defects, including limb abnormalities, skin scarring, and damage to the eyes and brain. The severity of these effects underscores the importance of vaccination and ensuring that women of childbearing age are immune to chickenpox before pregnancy.

Moreover, if a pregnant woman experiences chickenpox late in her pregnancy, there is a risk of the newborn developing neonatal varicella, which can be life-threatening. This condition typically occurs when the mother contracts chickenpox within five days before or two days after delivery. Infants with this illness may develop severe rashes, respiratory complications, and even a risk of death. Therefore, understanding the timing of the infection is crucial for expectant mothers and their healthcare providers.

Vaccination against chickenpox is a key preventive measure. Women planning to become pregnant should discuss their immunization status with their healthcare provider. The varicella vaccine is effective in preventing chickenpox, and women who are not immune are usually advised to receive the vaccine at least one month before attempting conception. This proactive approach significantly reduces the risk of adverse effects on the baby related to chickenpox infection during pregnancy.

In addition to the risks associated with maternal chickenpox infection, the impact on the baby can also extend to those who may have been exposed to the virus in utero. Babies born to mothers who had chickenpox can experience complications even if they appear healthy at birth. Therefore, ongoing monitoring and care for these infants are essential to address any potential health issues that may arise as they grow.

It is also important for parents to be aware of the emotional and psychological aspects of dealing with chickenpox during pregnancy. The anxiety surrounding the potential effects on the baby can be overwhelming. Support from healthcare professionals and open communication with family and friends can help alleviate some of these concerns. Education about the risks and benefits of vaccination, as well as understanding the nature of chickenpox, will empower parents to make informed decisions regarding their health and the health of their baby.

Vaccination Considerations for Pregnant Women

Vaccination during pregnancy is a critical consideration for expectant mothers, particularly regarding diseases like chickenpox. The varicella-zoster virus, which causes chickenpox, can lead to complications for the mother and the fetus if contracted during pregnancy. Pregnant women who have not had chickenpox or who have not been vaccinated are at a higher risk of severe outcomes if they contract the virus. Therefore, it is essential for parents-to-be to discuss their vaccination status with healthcare providers early in their prenatal care.

The timing and type of vaccination are crucial factors to consider. The varicella vaccine is a live attenuated vaccine, meaning it contains a weakened form of the virus. Because of this, it is not recommended for pregnant women to receive the vaccine while they are expecting. Instead, women who are planning to become pregnant should receive the vaccination at least a month before conception. This preventive strategy helps ensure that both the mother and the baby have protection against chickenpox and its potential complications.

In addition to the primary vaccination, understanding the potential risks of chickenpox during pregnancy is vital. If a pregnant woman contracts chickenpox, particularly in the first or second trimester, there is a risk of congenital varicella syndrome, which can result in severe birth defects. Furthermore, if a mother develops chickenpox shortly before or after delivery, the newborn may be at risk for serious complications, including a life-threatening form of chickenpox. Awareness of these risks underscores the importance of vaccination and preventive measures.

For those who are already pregnant and unsure of their varicella immunity, testing for immunity can be beneficial. A simple blood test can determine if a woman has the antibodies necessary to protect herself and her baby from chickenpox. If the test indicates a lack of immunity, healthcare providers may recommend close monitoring and additional precautions to minimize exposure to the virus, especially in environments where outbreaks may occur, such as schools or daycare centers.

It is essential for parents to stay informed about the myths and misconceptions surrounding chickenpox and its vaccination, especially concerning pregnancy. Many people may believe that chickenpox is not a serious illness or that vaccination is unnecessary. However, this perspective can be dangerous for pregnant women and their unborn children. Educating oneself about the real risks associated with chickenpox and the protective benefits of vaccination can empower parents to make informed decisions and foster a healthier future for their families.

Chapter 7: Chickenpox Recovery and Post-Infection Care

What to Expect During Recovery

During recovery from chickenpox, parents can expect a range of experiences as their child transitions from illness to health. The typical recovery period lasts around one to two weeks, during which the child will gradually see an improvement in symptoms. Initially, the fever and fatigue associated with the infection should subside, usually within a few days. As the body begins to heal, the skin lesions that characterize chickenpox will start to crust over, signaling that the contagious phase of the illness is coming to an end.

Parents should be vigilant about monitoring their child's symptoms during recovery. While the majority of children experience a mild course of the illness, some may develop complications such as bacterial infections of the skin, pneumonia, or neurological issues. Signs of complications can include increased redness or swelling around the blisters, difficulty breathing, or changes in behavior. If any alarming symptoms arise, timely consultation with a healthcare professional is crucial to ensure proper care and management.

Hydration and nutrition play a vital role in recovery. Parents should encourage their child to drink plenty of fluids to prevent dehydration, which can be exacerbated by fever and skin lesions. Balanced meals rich in vitamins and minerals can also support the immune system. Foods that are easy to swallow and gentle on the stomach, such as soups and smoothies, may be beneficial while the child is experiencing discomfort from mouth sores or lesions.

It is important to note that while recovery from chickenpox generally leads to lifelong immunity, some children may experience lingering effects, such as fatigue or skin sensitivity, for a short period after the rash has cleared. Encouraging rest and maintaining a calm environment can help facilitate a smoother transition back to normal activities. Parents should also be aware that the risk of developing shingles later in life remains for those who have had chickenpox, as the varicella-zoster virus can reactivate.

Finally, educating family members about the recovery process can help dispel myths and misconceptions surrounding chickenpox. Understanding that recovery is a natural progression and that most children will return to their regular routines without complications can ease parental concerns. Open discussions about chickenpox, its management, and recovery can empower parents and caregivers to provide the best care for their children and promote a supportive healing environment.

Post-Infection Skin Care

Post-infection skin care is a critical aspect of managing chickenpox, particularly as the visible signs of the illness begin to heal. After the blisters have crusted over and the fever has subsided, parents should focus on maintaining the integrity of the skin to promote healing and minimize the risk of scarring. The affected areas may still be sensitive, and gentle care is essential. Keeping the skin clean and moisturized can greatly aid in the recovery process. Use mild, fragrance-free soap during baths to avoid irritation, and consider applying an unscented lotion or cream to soothe the skin and reduce dryness.

It is important to monitor the healing process closely. Parents should watch for any signs of secondary infections, such as increased redness, swelling, or discharge from the blisters. These symptoms may indicate that bacteria have entered through the open sores. If such signs appear, seeking prompt medical attention is crucial to prevent complications. Additionally, be aware that some children may experience itchiness even after the blisters have healed. Over-the-counter antihistamines may help alleviate this discomfort, but it is essential to consult with a healthcare provider before administering any medication.

Sun exposure can also affect the healing skin, making it more susceptible to pigmentation changes and scarring. It is advisable to keep the child out of direct sunlight during the recovery period, especially if the skin is still healing. When outdoor activities are unavoidable, applying a broad-spectrum sunscreen with an appropriate SPF can help protect the skin. Additionally, wearing protective clothing can minimize sun exposure and further irritation, aiding in the overall healing process.

In some cases, scarring may occur, especially if the blisters were scratched or improperly treated. To reduce the chances of permanent marks, parents can consider using silicone gel sheets or topical treatments recommended by dermatologists. These products can help flatten and soften scars as the skin continues to heal. Furthermore, maintaining a healthy diet rich in vitamins A and C can support skin regeneration and overall recovery. Hydration is equally important, as it helps maintain skin elasticity and promotes healing.

Finally, emotional support during the post-infection period is essential. Children may feel self-conscious about their appearance as they recover from chickenpox, especially if there are visible marks on their skin. Open conversations about the healing process and reassurance that their skin will improve over time can help boost their confidence. Encouraging gentle, positive interactions and distractions, such as engaging in fun activities or hobbies, can also support emotional well-being during recovery. By providing comprehensive post-infection care, parents can help their children heal properly and restore their skin health effectively.

Monitoring for Long-term Effects

Monitoring for long-term effects after a chickenpox infection is crucial for ensuring the continued health and well-being of your child. While most children recover from chickenpox without any complications, some may experience long-term effects that parents should be aware of. These effects can range from skin problems, such as scarring from the rash, to more serious complications affecting the nervous system or other organs. Therefore, it is important to keep a close watch on your child's health during the recovery phase and beyond.

One common concern following chickenpox is the potential for scarring. The rash associated with chickenpox can leave marks on the skin, especially if blisters are scratched or not properly cared for. Parents should monitor the affected areas for signs of infection or unusual healing. Applying soothing lotions and keeping the skin moisturized can help minimize the risk of scarring. Consulting with a pediatrician can also provide guidance on post-infection skin care, ensuring that your child's skin recovers as smoothly as possible.

In addition to skin concerns, parents should be vigilant about neurological symptoms that could arise after a chickenpox infection. Although rare, conditions such as encephalitis or cerebellar ataxia can occur. Symptoms may include confusion, persistent headaches, or coordination issues. If your child exhibits any unusual behavior or neurological symptoms, it is essential to seek medical attention promptly. Early detection and intervention can significantly improve outcomes in such cases.

Furthermore, chickenpox can lead to complications in individuals with weakened immune systems. For parents of immunocompromised children, monitoring for signs of secondary infections or prolonged symptoms is vital. These children may face a higher risk of severe complications, making regular follow-ups with healthcare providers essential. Understanding your child's specific health needs and working closely with their medical team will help in managing any potential long-term effects effectively.

Lastly, it is important to educate yourself about the relationship between chickenpox and shingles, as the varicella-zoster virus that causes chickenpox can remain dormant in the body and reactivate later in life. Parents should be aware of the signs of shingles and the potential for their child to develop this condition in the future. Keeping an eye on your child's health history and discussing vaccination options with your healthcare provider can help in preventing shingles and mitigating long-term effects associated with chickenpox. By staying informed and proactive, you can help ensure your child's ongoing health and well-being.

Chapter 8: Chickenpox Myths and Misconceptions

Common Myths Debunked

One of the most pervasive myths surrounding chickenpox is that it is a harmless childhood illness that everyone must go through. While it is true that chickenpox is often milder in children compared to adults, it can still lead to significant complications, especially in certain populations. Parents should be aware that chickenpox can result in severe skin infections, pneumonia, and in rare cases, encephalitis, which is inflammation of the brain. Understanding that chickenpox is not merely a rite of passage can help parents make informed decisions about vaccination and prevention.

Another common misconception is that chickenpox vaccines are unnecessary because the disease is not life-threatening. This belief overlooks the critical fact that the vaccine not only reduces the risk of contracting chickenpox but also lessens the severity of the disease if a vaccinated person does become infected. Studies have shown that vaccinated individuals are less likely to experience the full-blown symptoms of chickenpox, such as fever and an extensive rash. Vaccination is a proactive measure that protects not only the individual but also vulnerable populations, such as infants and immunocompromised individuals who are at greater risk of severe illness.

Many parents also believe that natural remedies can effectively treat chickenpox symptoms without any medical intervention. While some home remedies, such as oatmeal baths and calamine lotion, can provide relief from itching and discomfort, they do not eliminate the virus or prevent complications. It is important for parents to understand that while these remedies may help manage symptoms, they should not replace medical advice or treatment. Consulting with a healthcare provider is crucial for ensuring proper care and monitoring of the infection.

There is a widespread belief that chickenpox is a childhood disease that cannot affect adults. In reality, adults who have never had chickenpox or have not been vaccinated can contract the virus, often experiencing more severe symptoms than children. Adults are at a higher risk for complications such as pneumonia and hospitalization. Parents should recognize that the importance of vaccination extends beyond childhood and that adults should also be informed about their vaccination status to prevent potential outbreaks in their families.

Finally, a significant misconception is that once a person has had chickenpox, they cannot experience any further health issues related to the virus. In fact, the varicella-zoster virus remains dormant in the body and can reactivate later in life, causing shingles. This painful condition can occur regardless of whether a person had chickenpox as a child. Parents should educate themselves about the connection between chickenpox and shingles, as well as the availability of vaccines that can prevent shingles in older adults. Understanding these myths and misconceptions is essential for comprehensive care and prevention strategies regarding chickenpox and its complications.

Understanding the Truth About Chickenpox

Understanding the truth about chickenpox is essential for parents as they navigate the complexities of this common childhood illness. Chickenpox, caused by the varicella-zoster virus, is characterized by an itchy rash, fever, and fatigue. While often seen as a rite of passage in childhood, understanding its implications is vital for proper management and prevention. Recognizing the symptoms early can help in reducing discomfort and preventing complications, especially in vulnerable populations such as infants, pregnant women, and immunocompromised individuals.

Vaccination plays a critical role in chickenpox prevention. The varicella vaccine, introduced in the mid-1990s, has significantly reduced the incidence of chickenpox and its associated complications. Parents should be aware that the vaccine not only prevents the illness but also lessens the severity of symptoms if a vaccinated child does contract the virus. It is recommended that children receive their first dose between 12 to 15 months of age and a second dose between 4 to 6 years. Understanding the vaccination schedule and its importance is crucial for protecting not just individual children but also the wider community.

Home remedies can provide relief from the uncomfortable symptoms of chickenpox. Parents can help their children manage itching and discomfort through various methods, such as oatmeal baths, calamine lotion, and antihistamines. Keeping nails trimmed and encouraging children not to scratch can prevent secondary infections. However, while these remedies can alleviate symptoms, they do not replace the need for medical advice or intervention in cases of severe symptoms or complications. Understanding when to seek medical help is an important aspect of caring for a child with chickenpox.

The impact of chickenpox varies significantly between children and adults. While children typically experience a mild course of the disease, adults are more likely to encounter severe symptoms and complications, such as pneumonia or encephalitis. This discrepancy underscores the importance of vaccination and awareness among parents, especially for teenagers and adults who may not have had chickenpox in childhood. Furthermore, chickenpox can pose serious risks during pregnancy, potentially leading to congenital varicella syndrome in the developing fetus. Understanding these risks can guide parents in making informed health decisions.

Myths and misconceptions about chickenpox abound, often leading to confusion and misinformation. One common myth is that chickenpox is a harmless childhood illness that does not require medical attention. In reality, complications can arise, particularly in at-risk populations. Additionally, the relationship between chickenpox and shingles is often misunderstood; the varicella-zoster virus remains dormant in the body after a chickenpox infection and can reactivate later in life as shingles. Educating parents about these aspects can help dispel myths and encourage proactive health measures, ensuring that children remain safe and healthy.

Educating Others

Educating others about chickenpox is crucial for fostering a well-informed community, as knowledge empowers parents to make effective decisions regarding prevention and care. Sharing accurate information about chickenpox, its symptoms, and how it spreads can help dispel common myths and misconceptions. For instance, many parents may believe that chickenpox is merely a childhood illness that children will inevitably contract. However, education emphasizes the importance of vaccination as a preventive measure, reducing the incidence of the disease and its potential complications.

When discussing chickenpox prevention, it is essential to highlight the effectiveness of the varicella vaccine. Parents should understand that the vaccine not only protects their children from contracting chickenpox but also contributes to herd immunity, which is vital for safeguarding those who cannot be vaccinated, such as immunocompromised individuals. By sharing personal experiences and credible resources, parents can encourage friends and family to prioritize vaccination, thereby reducing the overall prevalence of the virus in the community.

Home remedies for alleviating chickenpox symptoms are also an important topic for education. Parents can share effective strategies such as oatmeal baths or natural moisturizers to provide relief from itching and discomfort. Educating others on the proper care during an outbreak can significantly improve the quality of life for affected children and reduce the likelihood of secondary infections. This information can be particularly beneficial in community forums or parenting groups, where shared experiences can lead to collective learning and support.

The differences in chickenpox manifestations between adults and children are often overlooked. Educating others on these differences can help parents recognize when to seek medical attention. Adults tend to experience more severe symptoms and complications than children, making awareness crucial. By discussing these distinctions, parents can advocate for their children's health and encourage open conversations about the importance of monitoring symptoms and managing complications effectively.

Finally, addressing the impact of chickenpox on pregnancy is vital for expectant parents. Understanding the risks associated with chickenpox during pregnancy, including potential complications for both the mother and the unborn child, can lead to proactive measures. Parents can share information with those in their network about prenatal care and the importance of vaccination prior to conception. By educating others, parents not only protect their families but also contribute to a more informed community that values health and well-being.

Chapter 9: Chickenpox in Immunocompromised Individuals

Increased Risks

Increased risks associated with chickenpox extend beyond the immediate symptoms of the disease and can significantly impact various populations, particularly those who are immunocompromised, pregnant, or adults who contract the virus. While chickenpox is often considered a childhood illness, adults who lack immunity face a higher likelihood of severe complications. These can include pneumonia, encephalitis, and secondary bacterial infections, which necessitate close monitoring and potentially more aggressive treatment than typically required for children.

For parents, understanding the implications of chickenpox in children is crucial. While most children recover without serious issues, certain factors can elevate the risk of complications. Children with weakened immune systems due to conditions such as leukemia or those on immunosuppressive medications are at a heightened risk. Parents must be vigilant in identifying signs of complications early, as these children may require hospitalization or specialized care to manage their symptoms effectively.

Pregnant women who contract chickenpox face significant risks, both for themselves and their unborn children. The varicella virus can lead to congenital varicella syndrome, which can cause severe birth defects. Additionally, if a mother becomes infected close to her delivery date, there's a risk of neonatal varicella, a serious condition in newborns. Therefore, it is crucial for expectant mothers to be aware of their immunity status and to consult healthcare providers about vaccination or varicella zoster immune globulin if they are exposed to the virus.

Myths surrounding chickenpox often contribute to inadequate understanding of its risks. Some parents may believe that chickenpox is a harmless childhood rite of passage, but this perception can lead to complacency about vaccination and prevention strategies. The reality is that while mild cases do occur, the virus can lead to serious complications, particularly in vulnerable populations. Educating parents about the actual risks associated with chickenpox is essential for fostering informed decisions regarding vaccination and care.

Finally, the relationship between chickenpox and shingles underscores the importance of vaccination and prevention. A previous chickenpox infection can reactivate later in life as shingles, which carries its own set of risks and complications. Understanding this connection can help parents appreciate the long-term implications of chickenpox and the benefits of immunization for both children and adults. By prioritizing prevention and recognizing the increased risks associated with chickenpox, parents can better protect their families and contribute to community health.

Special Precautions

When addressing the topic of chickenpox, it is essential for parents to understand the special precautions necessary to protect their children and others in the community. Chickenpox is highly contagious and can spread easily through respiratory droplets or direct contact with the blisters of an infected person. Parents should ensure that their children avoid close contact with infected individuals, especially in environments such as schools and daycare centers, where the virus can spread rapidly. Keeping children home from school during the contagious period, which is typically from one to two days before the rash appears until all blisters have crusted over, is crucial in preventing outbreaks.

Vaccination remains one of the most effective strategies for chickenpox prevention. The varicella vaccine is recommended for children, adolescents, and adults who have not previously had the disease. Parents should verify their children's vaccination records and ensure they are up to date. In addition to individual protection, widespread vaccination contributes to herd immunity, which is vital for protecting those who cannot be vaccinated, such as infants and immunocompromised individuals. Parents should consult with their healthcare providers about the appropriate vaccination schedule and any potential side effects of the vaccine.

Home remedies can provide symptomatic relief for children suffering from chickenpox. Parents should consider using calamine lotion to soothe itching, and oatmeal baths can help alleviate discomfort from the rash. Keeping the child's nails trimmed short can prevent skin infections caused by scratching, while loose, breathable clothing can minimize irritation. It is important for parents to stay vigilant about maintaining hydration and providing a balanced diet during recovery, as the body needs adequate nutrition to heal effectively.

Parents should also be aware of the differences in chickenpox symptoms and complications that may arise in adults compared to children. Adults are more likely to experience severe symptoms and complications, such as pneumonia or encephalitis. Therefore, parents of adolescents and young adults should be particularly cautious and seek medical attention if symptoms worsen. Additionally, chickenpox can pose serious risks during pregnancy, including potential birth defects or complications for the mother. Pregnant women should consult with their healthcare providers regarding immunization and any necessary precautions.

Finally, it is important to dispel common myths and misconceptions surrounding chickenpox. Some parents may believe that chickenpox is a benign childhood illness that does not require serious attention; however, it can lead to complications, especially in vulnerable populations. Educating oneself about the nature of chickenpox, its transmission, and potential complications can empower parents to make informed decisions regarding prevention and care. Understanding the history and evolution of the chickenpox vaccine further highlights the importance of vaccination in reducing the incidence of this disease and its associated complications.

Treatment Considerations

Treatment considerations for chickenpox involve a multifaceted approach tailored to the age of the patient, the severity of symptoms, and any underlying health conditions. For most children, chickenpox is a mild disease that can be managed at home. Parents should focus on relieving uncomfortable symptoms such as itching and fever. Over-the-counter medications like acetaminophen can help manage fever, but aspirin should be avoided due to the risk of Reye's syndrome. Calamine lotion or antihistamines can effectively soothe itching. Maintaining a cool environment and encouraging loose, soft clothing can also provide relief, making the recovery process more comfortable for the child.

In cases where chickenpox occurs in adults, treatment considerations may differ due to the potential for more severe symptoms and complications. Adults are at a higher risk of experiencing pneumonia, hepatitis, and other serious conditions. It is essential for adult patients to monitor their symptoms closely and seek medical advice if complications arise. Antiviral medications, such as acyclovir, may be prescribed to reduce the severity and duration of the illness, especially if initiated within the first 24 hours of the rash appearing. Hydration and rest are equally crucial components of recovery for adults, as their bodies require more support to fight off the virus effectively.

For pregnant women, chickenpox poses unique risks to both the mother and the fetus. If a pregnant woman has not previously had chickenpox or received the vaccine, she should consult her healthcare provider immediately upon exposure to the virus. The treatment in this scenario may involve immunoglobulin therapy to prevent severe illness. The risks of congenital varicella syndrome, which can lead to serious birth defects, highlight the importance of vaccination before pregnancy. Parents should also be aware of the potential for passing the virus to newborns, which can result in severe complications if contracted in the first few weeks of life.

Individuals with compromised immune systems require specialized treatment considerations due to their increased vulnerability to severe chickenpox. These patients may need antiviral medications as a preventative measure, and their healthcare providers will likely monitor them more closely throughout the illness. Additional supportive care, such as nutritional support and careful management of any secondary infections, is crucial to help these individuals recover. Parents of immunocompromised children should ensure their child avoids exposure to infected individuals and consult medical professionals at the first sign of symptoms.

Addressing myths and misconceptions about chickenpox is essential in guiding treatment considerations. Many parents may believe that chickenpox is merely a childhood illness that is harmless; however, it can lead to serious complications in certain populations. Understanding the differences in treatment based on age and health condition can empower parents to seek appropriate care and make informed decisions about vaccinations. By fostering awareness and education about chickenpox, parents can better manage the illness within their families, ensuring a smoother recovery process for their children and themselves.

Chapter 10: The History and Evolution of the Chickenpox Vaccine

Development of the Vaccine

The development of the chickenpox vaccine marks a significant milestone in public health, transforming the way parents approach this common childhood illness. Chickenpox, caused by the varicella-zoster virus, was once considered a rite of passage for children, often resulting in discomfort and potential complications. The need for a vaccine became increasingly apparent as health professionals recognized the disease's impact on both children and adults, leading to the first steps toward creating a safe and effective immunization.

In the late 1960s, researchers began to explore the possibility of a vaccine after observing that individuals who had contracted a mild form of varicella were less likely to experience severe disease later in life. This observation laid the groundwork for the development of the live attenuated vaccine, which uses a weakened form of the virus to stimulate an immune response without causing the disease itself. The innovative approach aimed to provide immunity while minimizing the risks associated with chickenpox, particularly in vulnerable populations such as immunocompromised individuals and pregnant women.

The first successful chickenpox vaccine was licensed for use in Japan in 1986, followed by its introduction in the United States in 1995. The vaccine demonstrated impressive efficacy, reducing the incidence of chickenpox by more than 90% in vaccinated populations. As the vaccine became widely available, public health officials observed a marked decline in hospitalizations and complications associated with chickenpox. This success not only highlighted the importance of vaccination in preventing disease but also underscored the need for continued education and outreach to encourage immunization among parents.

Ongoing research and development have further refined the chickenpox vaccine, leading to the establishment of routine vaccination schedules for children. The two-dose regimen, recommended for children at ages 12-15 months and 4-6 years, ensures long-lasting immunity and significantly reduces the likelihood of shingles later in life. This is particularly crucial, as shingles, a reactivation of the varicella-zoster virus, can occur in adults who had chickenpox as children. The relationship between the two conditions emphasizes the importance of vaccination not only for immediate protection but also for long-term health benefits.

As parents consider the implications of vaccination, it is essential to address myths and misconceptions surrounding the chickenpox vaccine. Concerns about vaccine safety and the necessity of immunization are common, yet extensive research supports the vaccine's safety profile. Understanding the historical context and scientific advancements behind the chickenpox vaccine empowers parents to make informed decisions for their children's health. By prioritizing vaccination, families play a crucial role in safeguarding their children against chickenpox and its potential complications, fostering a healthier future for all.

Historical Impact of Vaccination

The historical impact of vaccination, particularly in relation to chickenpox, is profound and has shaped public health strategies over the decades. Before the introduction of the chickenpox vaccine in the mid-1990s, the disease was a common childhood illness that affected nearly every child by the age of 15. While chickenpox is often considered a mild disease, its complications can be severe, especially in immunocompromised individuals and adults. The widespread implementation of the vaccine has significantly reduced the incidence of chickenpox, leading to fewer cases of hospitalization and complications associated with the disease.

The evolution of the chickenpox vaccine began with the recognition of the varicella-zoster virus as the causative agent of the disease. In

Japan, researchers developed the first live attenuated vaccine against chickenpox in the 1970s, which was later introduced in the United States in 1995. This marked a critical turning point in public health, as the vaccine not only protected children from chickenpox but also contributed to herd immunity, reducing transmission rates across the entire population. By vaccinating children, communities could lower the overall prevalence of the virus, benefiting those who were unable to receive the vaccine due to medical reasons.

The impact of the chickenpox vaccination program has been notable in terms of public health outcomes. Since its introduction, the incidence of chickenpox has dropped by more than 90 percent in vaccinated populations. This decline has translated into a significant reduction in healthcare costs associated with treating chickenpox-related complications. Parents have been relieved of the burden of managing severe cases in their children, and the number of hospitalizations due to chickenpox has dramatically decreased. The success of this vaccine has also paved the way for further research and development of vaccines against other childhood diseases.

Additionally, the relationship between chickenpox and shingles highlights the importance of vaccination in preventing both diseases. When a person contracts chickenpox, the varicella-zoster virus remains dormant in the nervous system and can reactivate later in life as shingles. Vaccination against chickenpox not only protects against the initial infection but also reduces the risk of developing shingles later on. This dual protection underscores the long-term benefits of vaccination for individuals and communities alike.

Despite the successes associated with the chickenpox vaccine, myths and misconceptions persist, influencing parental decisions regarding vaccination. Educating parents about the historical impact of vaccination can help dispel fears and encourage informed choices. Understanding that widespread vaccination has led to a significant decrease in chickenpox cases, complications, and associated healthcare costs can empower parents to protect their children and contribute to public health efforts. By acknowledging the history and effectiveness of chickenpox vaccination, parents can make better decisions that ensure the health and safety of their families and communities.

Future Directions in Vaccine Research

Future directions in vaccine research for chickenpox hold promise for enhancing prevention strategies and improving overall public health outcomes. As the understanding of the varicella-zoster virus deepens, scientists are exploring innovative approaches that could further reduce the incidence of chickenpox and its complications. This includes the development of more effective vaccines, possible combination vaccines that include protection against shingles, and research into alternative delivery mechanisms that could simplify immunization.

One area of focus is the improvement of current chickenpox vaccines, particularly the live attenuated varicella vaccine. Researchers are investigating ways to enhance the vaccine's efficacy and duration of immunity. This might involve refining the viral strains used in the vaccine or altering the formulation to stimulate a stronger immune response. Enhanced vaccines could potentially reduce breakthrough infections and minimize the need for booster doses, making vaccination more accessible and convenient for families.

Another exciting avenue is the exploration of combination vaccines that would protect against multiple diseases in a single shot. By combining the chickenpox vaccine with vaccines for other childhood illnesses, such as measles, mumps, and rubella, researchers aim to increase vaccination rates and simplify the immunization schedule for parents. This approach not only saves time but also reduces the number of injections children receive, making the overall vaccination experience less daunting.

In addition to vaccine formulation and delivery, ongoing studies are examining the long-term effects of chickenpox vaccination on community immunity and the epidemiology of the disease.

Understanding how widespread vaccination impacts the incidence of chickenpox and shingles, especially in adults who were vaccinated as children, is crucial. This research could inform public health policies and vaccination recommendations, ensuring that the benefits of vaccination are maximized while minimizing the risks associated with varicella-zoster reactivation.

Finally, as vaccine technology continues to evolve, researchers are also looking into new platforms, such as mRNA vaccines, which have gained attention due to their effectiveness in the fight against COVID-19. Exploring these innovative technologies could lead to breakthroughs in the development of next-generation chickenpox vaccines that offer improved safety profiles and efficacy. By staying at the forefront of vaccine research, scientists aim to provide parents with even more effective tools to prevent chickenpox and its associated complications, ultimately leading to healthier futures for children and communities alike.

Chapter 11: Chickenpox and its Relation to Shingles

Understanding the Connection

The connection between chickenpox and various health implications is critical for parents seeking to navigate this common childhood illness. Chickenpox, caused by the varicella-zoster virus, primarily affects children but can also have significant effects on adults and individuals with weakened immune systems. Understanding these connections can empower parents to make informed decisions regarding prevention, treatment, and care. Recognizing the symptoms of chickenpox, such as an itchy rash, fever, and fatigue, is the first step in addressing this illness effectively.

Vaccination plays a pivotal role in preventing chickenpox and its potential complications. The varicella vaccine has been instrumental in reducing the incidence of chickenpox in children, leading to a decrease in related hospitalizations and complications. Parents should be aware of the recommended vaccination schedule, which typically includes two doses: the first at 12 to 15 months of age and the second at 4 to 6 years. Understanding the impact of vaccination not only protects individual children but also contributes to community immunity, safeguarding those who cannot be vaccinated due to medical reasons.

Home remedies can provide relief for children suffering from chickenpox symptoms, helping to alleviate discomfort during the illness. Oatmeal baths, for instance, can soothe itchy skin, while calamine lotion can be applied to rash areas to reduce irritation. Parents should also ensure that their child remains hydrated and receives adequate rest to support recovery. However, it is essential to differentiate between home remedies and medical treatments, as certain symptoms may require professional evaluation, particularly if complications arise.

The relationship between chickenpox and shingles is another important aspect for parents to understand. Once a person has had chickenpox, the virus remains dormant in the body and can reactivate later in life, resulting in shingles. This condition can be particularly painful and may lead to complications, especially in older adults. Parents should educate themselves about the signs of shingles and consider vaccination options available for older children and adults to reduce the risk of this painful condition later in life.

Finally, it is crucial to dispel myths and misconceptions surrounding chickenpox. Many parents may believe that chickenpox is a harmless rite of passage or that natural infection is better than vaccination. However, this perspective overlooks the potential risks, including severe complications that can arise in otherwise healthy children and the impact on immunocompromised individuals. By understanding the facts about chickenpox, its prevention through vaccination, and the importance of proper care during infection, parents can take proactive steps to protect their children and contribute to a healthier community.

Shingles Risks in Adults

Shingles, also known as herpes zoster, is a significant risk for adults who have previously contracted chickenpox. After a person recovers from chickenpox, the varicella-zoster virus remains dormant in the nervous system and can reactivate years later, leading to shingles. This condition typically manifests as a painful rash that can appear anywhere on the body, often following a dermatome, or a specific area of skin supplied by a single spinal nerve. The risk of developing shingles increases with age, making it particularly important for parents to understand the implications of chickenpox in their own health as well as their children's.

The incidence of shingles is notably higher in adults, especially those over the age of 50. Factors such as stress, weakened immune systems, and certain medical conditions can increase susceptibility to the reactivation of the virus. Parents should be aware that while chickenpox is often milder in children, the potential for shingles poses a more serious health risk in adulthood. Understanding this risk is essential for informed decision-making about vaccination and preventive measures for both themselves and their children.

Vaccination plays a crucial role in reducing the risk of shingles. The shingles vaccine is recommended for adults aged 50 and older, regardless of whether they recall having chickenpox. Administering the varicella vaccine to children not only helps prevent chickenpox but also lowers the risk of shingles later in life. Parents should consult with their healthcare providers about vaccination schedules to ensure optimal protection against both chickenpox and shingles.

In addition to vaccination, recognizing the symptoms of shingles is vital for prompt treatment. Early signs include localized pain, tingling, or itching, often accompanied by a rash that develops into fluid-filled blisters. If parents or adults experience these symptoms, seeking medical advice can lead to timely intervention, which may include antiviral medications that can reduce the severity and duration of the outbreak. Understanding these symptoms can lead to better management of the condition and minimize complications.

Finally, it is essential to address the myths and misconceptions surrounding shingles and its relationship with chickenpox. Many believe that shingles can be contracted from someone with chickenpox, but it is actually the reactivation of a previous infection. Parents should educate themselves and their families about the realities of shingles, fostering a better understanding of the condition and encouraging proactive measures. This knowledge not only helps in managing their own health but also equips them to support their children in navigating the risks associated with chickenpox and its aftermath.

Prevention Strategies for Shingles

Prevention strategies for shingles largely revolve around understanding the connection between chickenpox and shingles, as well as taking proactive measures to reduce the risk of transmission and infection. Shingles, also known as herpes zoster, occurs when the varicella-zoster virus, which causes chickenpox, reactivates in the body. For parents, educating themselves and their children about the importance of vaccination against chickenpox is crucial. The varicella vaccine not only protects against chickenpox but also significantly reduces the likelihood of developing shingles later in life. Ensuring that children receive the vaccine according to the recommended schedule is one of the most effective strategies for preventing shingles.

In addition to vaccination, parents can take steps to minimize the risk of exposure to the varicella-zoster virus, especially in environments where children may come into contact with infected individuals. This is particularly important during outbreaks of chickenpox in schools or community settings. Encouraging good hygiene practices, such as regular handwashing and avoiding sharing personal items, can help reduce the spread of the virus. Parents should also be vigilant about monitoring for symptoms of chickenpox, including rashes and fever, and seek medical advice promptly if they suspect their child may be infected.

For families with immunocompromised individuals or those who are pregnant, additional precautions are necessary. It is essential to limit exposure to individuals who have active chickenpox or shingles, as these infections can pose serious risks for those with weakened immune systems. Parents should communicate with schools and caregivers about the importance of keeping potentially contagious individuals away from vulnerable family members. In cases where a family member has shingles, maintaining a safe distance and practicing diligent hygiene can help protect others in the home.

Home remedies can also play a role in managing symptoms and preventing complications associated with chickenpox, which can indirectly help in reducing the risk of shingles. Parents should consider soothing treatments for chickenpox symptoms, such as oatmeal baths, calamine lotion, and cool compresses, to alleviate discomfort and minimize the severity of the infection. Ensuring that children receive proper care during their chickenpox infection can decrease the likelihood of complications that could trigger the reactivation of the virus later in life.

Finally, it is essential for parents to address myths and misconceptions surrounding chickenpox and shingles. Understanding that shingles can occur even in individuals who had mild chickenpox as children can help parents take the virus seriously. Educating themselves and their children about the importance of preventive measures and the significance of the varicella vaccine can empower families to make informed decisions. By fostering a proactive approach to prevention, parents can significantly contribute to the health and well-being of their children, reducing the risk of both chickenpox and shingles in their family.

www.ingramcontent.com/pod-product-compliance
Lightning Source LLC
Chambersburg PA
CBHW061526250726
48657CB00005B/2102